For our families and friends:
thank you for helping us to live life well.

Introduction

Friendship is born
at that moment
when one person
says to another,
"What, you too?"

C.S. Lewis

For us, that moment came back in 1984, when we met at Oxford University. Fast forward to 2021 and we are still firm friends, although we live on opposite sides of the Atlantic, in Buffalo, New York and Cardiff, Wales.

Four years ago, we decided to start a blog to help us to connect more often. We called it Staircase 917 – from the location of our rooms at Pembroke College – and there we talk about the small steps we can all take to make a difference in the world and to ourselves. This book brings together some of those ideas and more, as a year-round reference for ways to live life well.

With the help of our dear friend and talented designer and photographer, Cristina, we have written the book against the backdrop of the Covid-19 pandemic, in three different cities on two continents. Living life as well as possible has never seemed so important and we hope you will enjoy these ideas to help us all do so.

Sam and Claire
www.staircase917.com

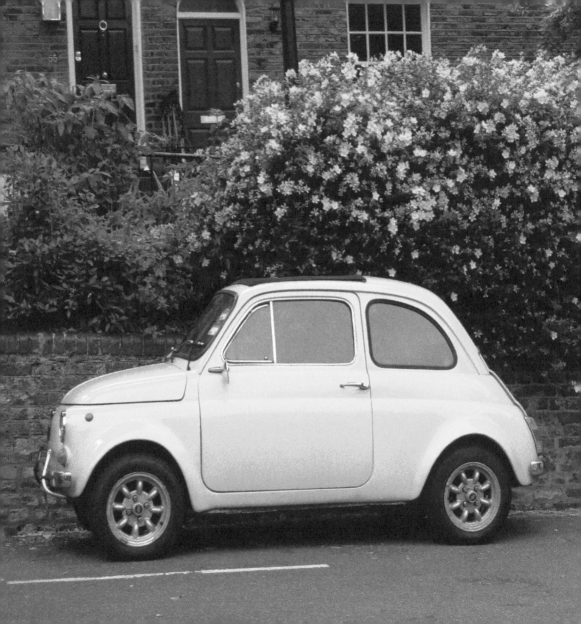

Little Ideas for January

It is never too late to be
what you might have been.

George Eliot

January is an interesting mix of a month. It's a brand new year, with its sense of hope and renewal, and yet it can be grey and damp or bitterly cold with the prospect of weeks of winter ahead. So as the calendar turns we find ourselves wanting to capture some sunshine, and what better way than in the form of citrus?

There are many links between citrus and well-being. Not only are oranges, lemons, kumquats, limes and grapefruits full of Vitamin C, helping to ward off or shorten colds and keep skin healthy, they are also rich in potassium and roughage, and good for your heart and digestion. They release their sugar energy slowly, keeping you feeling full for longer, and they help release the iron in other foods.

Citrus fruits also have a lot of water content and sometimes we struggle to drink enough, especially this time of year, cooped up in a dry, heated home. So what better than some

> The aroma of citrus fruits increases levels of serotonin and reduces those of stress hormones, promoting both happiness and calm.

tangy lemon-infused water to begin the day? Or a nice, sweet, juicy orange as a hydrating snack – alongside a square or two of iron-rich dark chocolate?

There's nothing like deeply breathing in the scent of a fresh orange, lemon or grapefruit. There are several studies on their mood-boosting properties. Add the warm, bright hues of citrus fruits, and you have a strong association with happy sun-filled days. So make a resolution in these cold, dark winter months to lose yourself for a few moments each day in the heady scent of citrus; and taste a little happiness and sunshine!

Resolve to keep happy.

Helen Keller

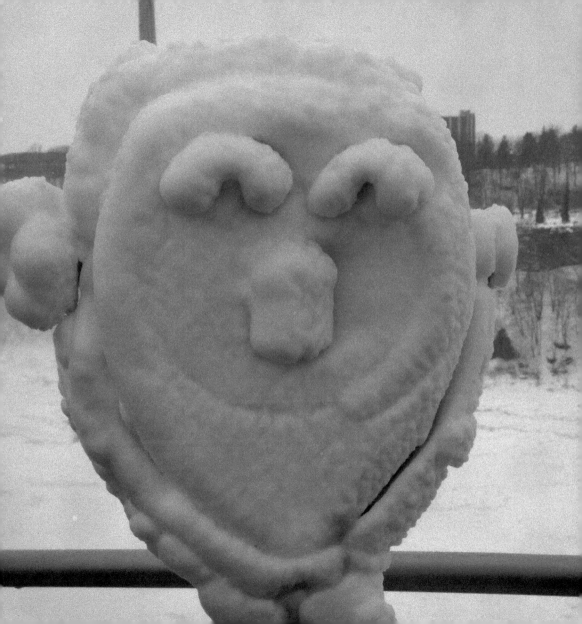

January is traditionally the time for resolutions. And by February they've often gone by the wayside. It can be hard to keep resolutions if they are too big or too focused on an outcome, rather than the process of getting there. We have found that the key is making one small decision at a time. For example instead of setting a weight loss target, try focusing on one meal at a time, deciding to make each plate small, natural and simple. A friend found success by imagining at each meal how a monk might eat, enjoying one small plate only, eating slowly and relishing each bite. Or instead of setting a fitness goal, decide to take out your bike each day, and enjoy the ride!

Walk in the sunshine. Jump in the ocean. Say the truth that you're carrying in your heart like a hidden treasure. Be silly. Be kind. Be weird. There is no time for anything else.
Anthony Hopkins

Our resolution this year is simply to enjoy the process of living life as well as we can. Here are some ideas to get started, and we hope you'll find more in the pages to come.

Happy new year!

- Fill your basket with citrus (p 8)
- Give up clutter, one thing at a time (p 16)
- Do an unexpected kindness for someone (p 24)
- Enjoy a bite of chocolate (p 36)
- Help a bee (p 44)
- Make lavender lemonade (p 52)
- Leave your lawn unmown (p 60)
- Go for a hike and help a charity (p 65)
- Play an online game and feed the world (p 76)
- Smile (p 80)
- Focus on your breathing (p 88)
- Roast some chestnuts (p 100)

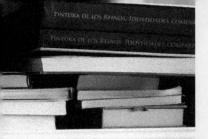
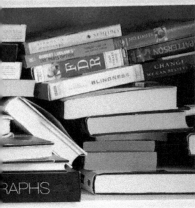
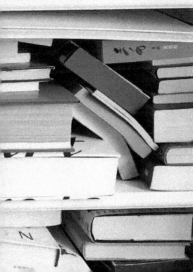

Little Ideas for February

Out of the clutter,
bring simplicity.

Albert Einstein

This is the time of year when, after indulging in pancakes and with any luck, Valentine chocolates, the question becomes what to give up – whether for Lent, or just general well-being.

Here are a couple of ideas beyond letting go of your most loved foods...

Give up clutter

Removing clutter from our homes has many health and psychological benefits, reducing anxiety, and bringing order and calm. Decluttering itself can seem overwhelming, though. We have found it helpful to start small. If you do use Lent as your opportunity, consider choosing just one thing a day to let go of and put it in a box. Then, when Lent is over, take the box to a thrift or charity shop. If you can enlist others in your home to fill up a box as well, so much the better.

Give up your mobile phone at night

If you use your phone as an alarm clock, it can be easy to get into the habit of checking news and texts and emails immediately before switching the light out, and then again as soon as you wake up. This means you are not transitioning restfully in and out of the day, but there's something about that mobile phone that is somehow addictive. Try a digital detox for the first and last hour of each day by charging your phone overnight in another room, and going back to a regular alarm clock, or a daylight clock for a more natural wake-up call.

'February' comes from the Latin word for purification, though the Anglo-Saxons called it cake month!

Winter is a season of recovery and preparation.

Paul Theroux

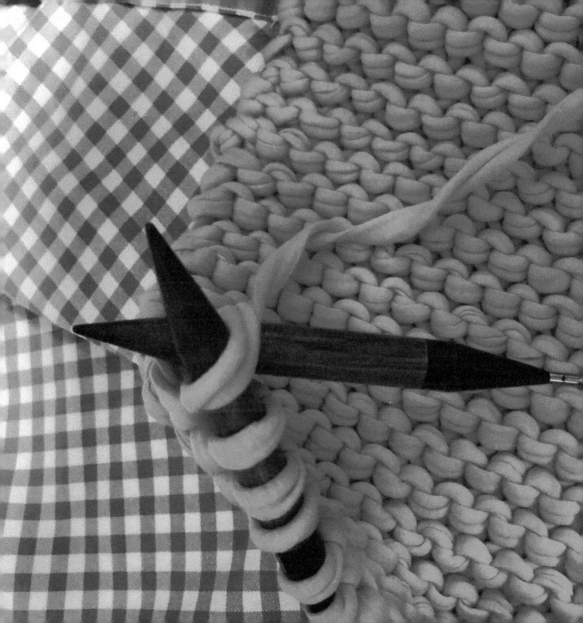

LEMON GINGER TONIC

In the cold, dark days of February, when the elements outside and heating inside can damage our skin and make us more susceptible to colds, it's important to stay hydrated. Try adding interest and nourishment to water by infusing it with berries, cucumber or mint. Or, for a warming detox that helps to ward off winter ills, here is a simple lemon ginger tonic.

Makes two servings

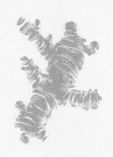

Ingredients
2 cups (500 ml) of water
Half a lemon, sliced
1 in (3cm) piece of ginger, sliced
1 teaspoon honey, or to taste

Method
Boil water in a saucepan and remove from the heat
Add the lemon and ginger
Steep for five minutes, then strain
Pour into a mug and stir in honey to sweeten

Optional
Add a shot of whiskey or rum for a soothing hot toddy

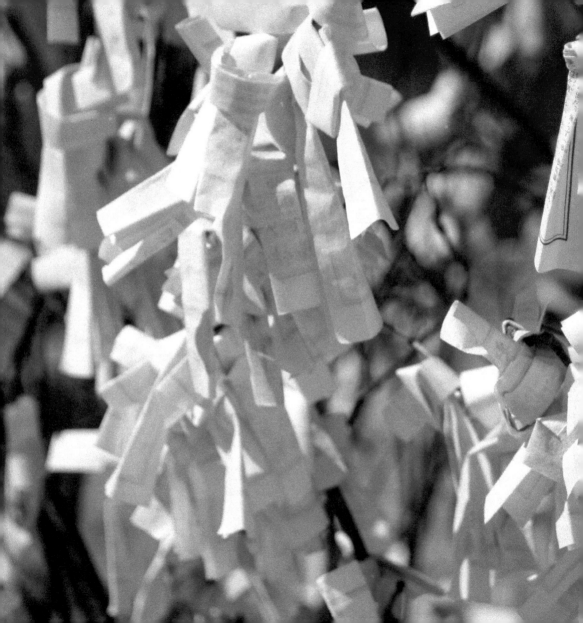

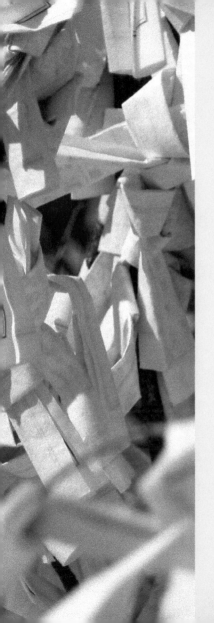

Little Ideas for March

Do the little things.

St David

March begins with the feast of St David, the patron saint of Wales. St David was a Celtic monk who lived a simple, gentle life and encouraged his followers to be joyful and to '*do the little things*' – acts of kindness which are within our reach every day.

Studies in positive psychology have shown that kindness is contagious - or 'generally reciprocal' as Dr Johnson put it. This is sometimes called the ripple effect, and research has shown that even one small gesture may inspire someone to go on to make a bigger commitment, perhaps to helping others by volunteering or getting involved in a local cause.

Here are some very simple gestures of kindness that enhance wellbeing day by day. These come from Action for Happiness, whose mission is to help people take action for a happier world. You can find many more ideas in the free calendars on their website, actionforhappiness.org.

- Send a positive message to someone you can't be with

- Give someone your place in line

- Share an encouraging news story

- Make someone smile

- Say hello to someone who lives nearby

- Give away your change

- Pay a compliment

- Offer to help

In one study, people who carried out six small acts of kindness in a day were still feeling increased levels of happiness six weeks later. And so it's true that helping others helps us, too.

I would always rather be happy than dignified.

Charlotte Brontë

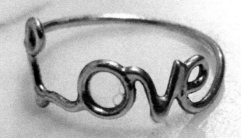

The 20th of March, the vernal equinox and the first day of spring, is also the International Day of Happiness. The United Nations launched this day in 2013, based on an idea from Bhutan, where Gross National Happiness is valued more than Gross National Product. The International Day of Happiness recognizes that progress should help to increase human wellbeing, and not just economics. All 193 member nations of the UN have adopted a resolution to give happiness greater priority. In the words of Ban-Ki Moon, then Secretary General of the UN, *the pursuit of happiness is a serious business.*

I want to be happy, But I won't be happy,
Till I make you happy, too.

Irving Caesar & Vincent Yeoman

According to Action for Happiness, while our genes account for about half of our predisposition to happiness, our circumstances, such as income and environment, account for only 10%. The other 40% comes from the choices we make and the actions we take every day.

By engaging in those little acts of kindness we mentioned on page 25, we are activating the parts of our brains that are associated with pleasure, social connection and trust of each other. This releases endorphins and increases not only the happiness of others, but also our own.

In our personal pursuit of happiness, we always mark the month of March and St David's Day with a bunch of daffodils, the national flower of Wales. Daffodils somehow bring a burst of sunshine into any room, and as the season begins to turn from winter to spring, it's the perfect time to wish for us all the very thing that daffodils symbolize: happy memories and happy new beginnings!

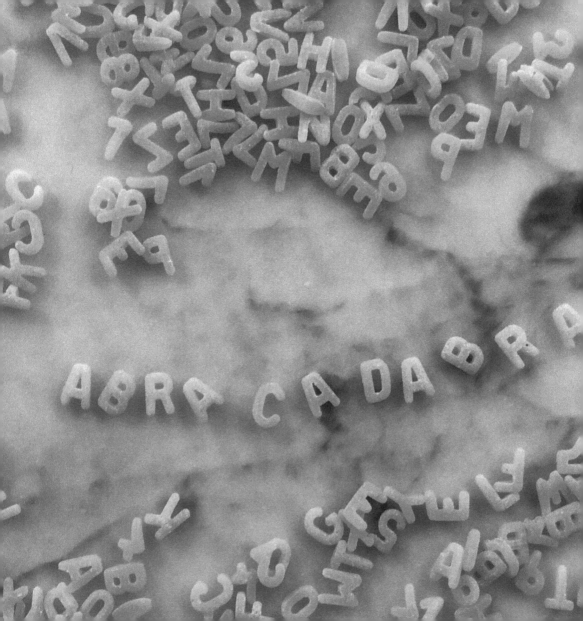

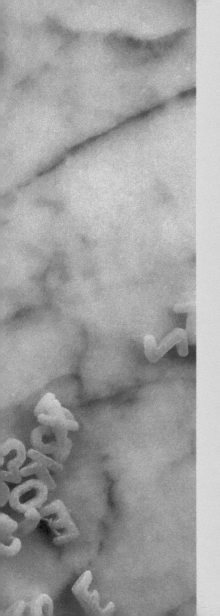

Little Ideas for April

Life is a combination of magic and pasta.

Federico Fellini

The 6th of April marks Italy's national carbonara day, and it's a pasta dish we love, so this month we're going to talk about food. Federico Fellini's many films include *La Dolce Vita* (*the sweet life*) and we believe food can be an important part of living the good life, bringing us pleasure when we share it. Cooking for people we care about is a simple act of love, and seeing others enjoy something we've made for them is one of life's great joys.

Our memories of food and meals can be very vivid; psychologists think this may be because they often involve all five of our senses. Foods can also have a direct effect on our mood, as we all know if we get grumpy when we're hungry. Perhaps it's no surprise to learn that the carbohydrates in pasta increase the body's production of serotonin, which helps us feel a sense of well-being and contentment.

Other foods that will boost your mood:

- Oily fish: good for brain function thanks to Omega 3
- Oats: release energy slowly to keep us going
- Bananas: contain magnesium and potassium and can help reduce sleeplessness and anxiety
- Lentils: help regulate our blood sugar
- Spinach: rich in iron, which helps in transporting oxygen around the body. It also contains vitamin K which is important for bone health

William Shakespeare, born in April 1564, mentions food in every one of his plays, and coined phrases including 'salad days', 'eaten out of house and home' and 'the world's your oyster'.

All you need is love. But a little chocolate now and then doesn't hurt.

Charles Schultz

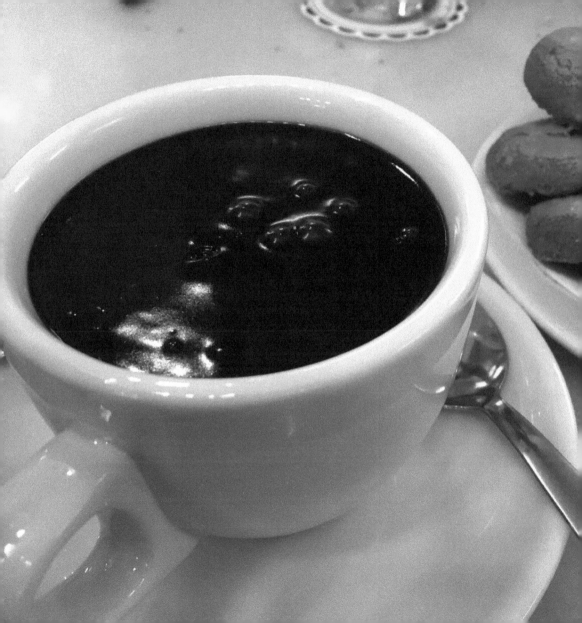

CHOCOLATE LIME THINS

Perhaps the most popular feel-good food of all is chocolate, eaten and given when we want to celebrate or commiserate. Once known as the 'food of the gods', its use stretches back for 4000 years. The first chocolate bar was sold in 1847 and today more than $75 billion is spent worldwide on chocolate every year.

We shouldn't feel too guilty about enjoying it, though, as it contains magnesium and other minerals that regulate brain chemistry and cause a burst of contentment.

Ingredients
5½ oz (150g) plain chocolate
1¾ oz (50g) dark brown or Demerara sugar
½ teaspoon lime oil

Method
Melt the chopped plain chocolate in a bowl
over a pan of simmering water
Remove from the heat and stir in the sugar
and lime oil

Pour onto a sheet of 12in x 15in baking
parchment paper and spread it out a little
Top with another sheet and spread again
through the paper with a spatula or palette
knife into a thin layer
Chill for 40 minutes, peel off paper and slice
into squares

Ideal to serve with coffee or ice-cream

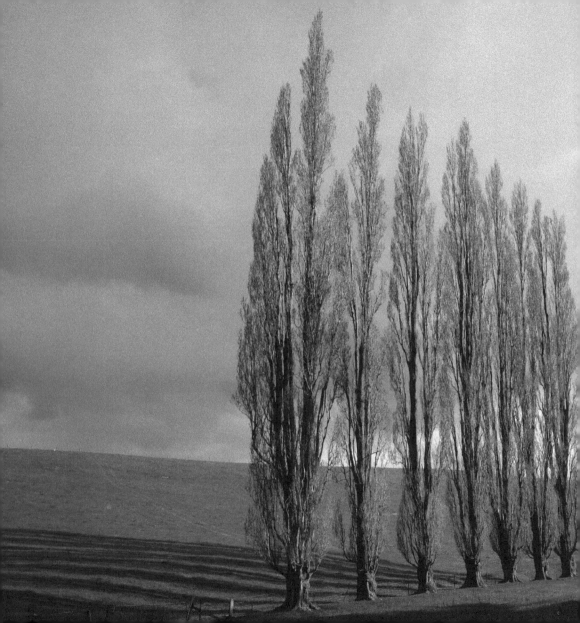

Little Ideas for May

March winds and
April showers,
bring forth
May flowers.
Proverb

Spring has finally sprung. It's lovely to be able to get outside, walk in the park and breathe in the fresh air – the perfect thing to add a touch of happiness to the day.

It's the season for planting, too. Depending on where you live, you may still have a few frosts early in the month, but while it's still chilly it's the perfect time to start growing some herbs. They're easy to cultivate even on a windowsill - especially sage, parsley, oregano, mint and basil. If you enjoy baking, fresh herbs add extra deliciousness to cheese scones. Or you might like to chop them finely and mix into room-temperature butter; or infuse a vinaigrette.

Herbs are quick to grow, so if you find yourself with a surplus, preserve some by tying in small bunches and hanging upside down in a cool, well-ventilated room for a few days to dry, then crumble and store in jars. Or freeze them in ice cube trays, in either water or olive oil.

Once it begins to warm up you can start to plant seedlings outdoors or sow seeds for late summer harvests. Look for planting calendars online from the *Farmers' Almanac* or the Royal Horticultural Society. If you don't have a garden of your own, consider joining or volunteering in a community garden, where you can make new friends, learn new skills, grow and share produce, and benefit others too.

Where we are, outdoor farmers markets start up in May. There's nothing like getting up early, cup of coffee in hand, chatting with the growers and browsing the stalls for fresh flowers and produce, home-baked bread and locally brewed beverages. A wonderful start to a spring weekend!

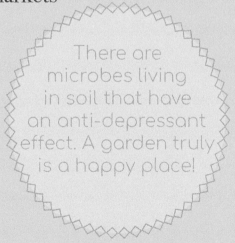

There are microbes living in soil that have an anti-depressant effect. A garden truly is a happy place!

To plant a garden is to believe in tomorrow.

Audrey Hepburn

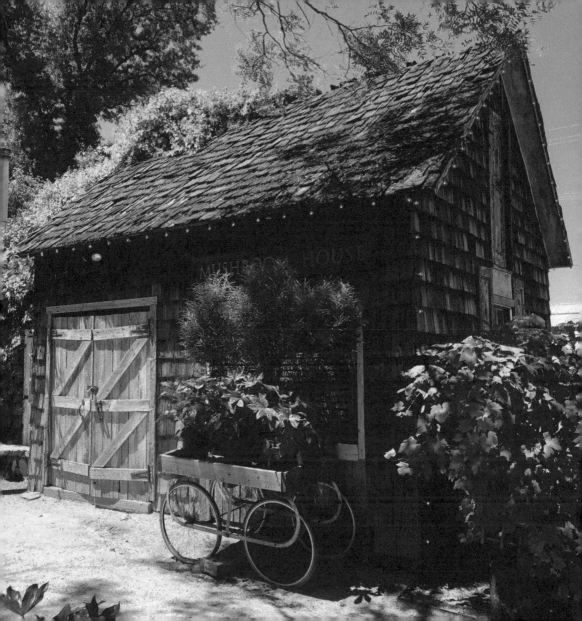

May 20th is World Bee Day, when we celebrate the vital role of pollinators like bees in ensuring flowers and plants thrive.

As the weather warms up, bees may start flagging in the heat. If you find a bee that is struggling, lift it out of harm's way onto a nearby flower so it can feed and get energy from the nectar. If there are no bee-friendly flowers nearby and you're sure it's not just resting, you can offer it a simple solution of sugar and water. Mix two tablespoons of white, granulated sugar with one tablespoon of water and place on a spoon for the bee to reach.

According to the United Nations, about 40% of the world's pollinators are under threat of extinction. Yet they are all so critical to us for pollinating the crops that keep us alive! So if each of us can help even one small bee recover, we'll be making a difference to us all.

Of course, without bees we wouldn't have honey*. Honey has been used in medicinal substances since ancient Egyptian times and has several benefits:

- It is rich in anti-oxidants and may help to lower blood pressure and cholesterol
- Applied to the skin, it can help heal wounds or burns
- It is a soothing remedy for coughs and sore throats

And of course, it is delicious! If for no other reason, that's worth helping a bee on its way. As Piglet understood well, all good friends need some honey sometimes.

"I don't feel very much like Pooh today," said Pooh.
"There, there," said Piglet.
"I'll bring you tea and honey until you do."

*please note, honey should never be given to children under one year old

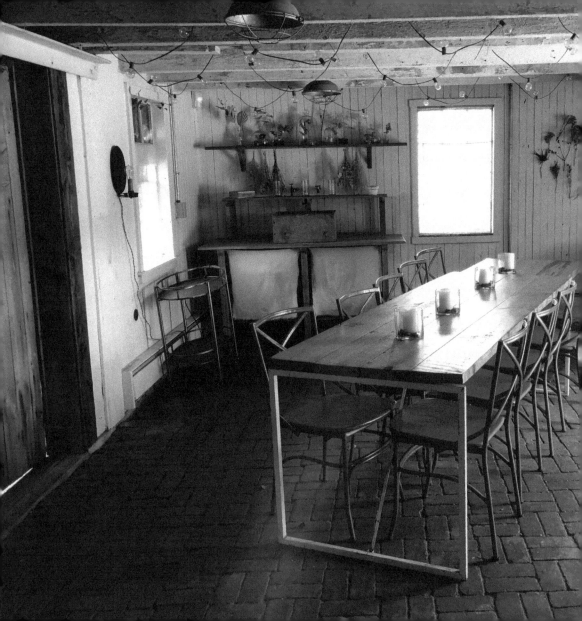

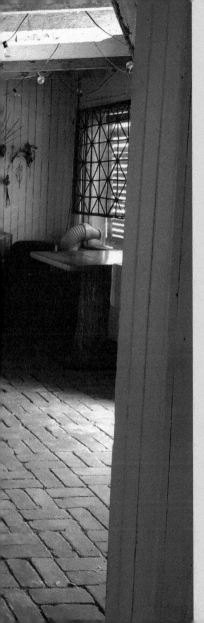

Little Ideas for June

We cannot have a perfect
life without friends.

Dante Alighieri

We've chosen this month to celebrate friends. Our female friendships are grounded in empathy and are especially important for emotional support in anxious times. And recent times have been rather stressful for us all in different ways.

In their book *Burnout*, twin sisters Emily and Amelia Nagoski talk about the effects of stress on our bodies and ways to overcome it in order to live a happier life. Three things that resonate with us:

- Wellbeing is not a state of being or state of mind, but a state of action
- The cure for stress is not caring for ourselves so much as caring for each other
- One effective way to do this is to give someone a hug

For those times when we cannot give our friends an actual hug, the charity KidsPeace has developed a virtual hug.

Their focus is children in need, but any friends can use this to help both experience the benefits in a time of isolation:

- Give yourself a self-hug. Cross your arms and hold your upper-arms, to create the physical sensation of hugging someone
- Take some slow deep breaths, to help slow your heart rate and give the calming effect of a hug
- Tell your friend something nice or reassuring, as a positive counter-balance to upsetting times

It's a simple idea. But however and whenever you can do it, consider giving a friend a twenty-second hug.

A hug releases oxytocin, a hormone that communicates love, belonging and trust. Studies show that this effect is particularly strong in women.

Women are like teabags, you don't know how
strong they are until you put them
in hot water.

Eleanor Roosevelt

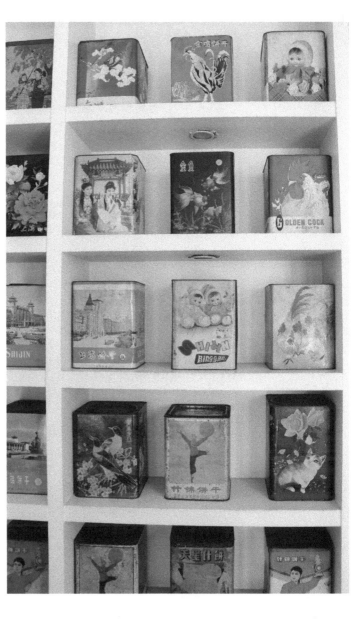

Kin Loch
Lavender Lemonade

As we head into longer summer days, and
lavender comes into bloom, what nicer way
to enjoy it than a glass of lemonade with our
friends. This recipe comes from Kin Loch
Farmstead in Sanborn, New York:
www.kinlochfarmstead.com

Ingredients
1 cup (225 g) white sugar
1 tbsp lavender buds (fresh or dry)
1½ cups (375 ml) fresh squeezed lemon juice
2 cups (500 ml) boiling water
Approximately 2 cups (500 ml) cold water
and ice to taste

Method
Put the sugar in a bowl
Add the lavender buds
Add the boiling water
Stir and let steep for 15-30 minutes
Strain everything into a large pitcher
Add the lemon juice, and stir
Add cold water and ice until the taste
is to your liking

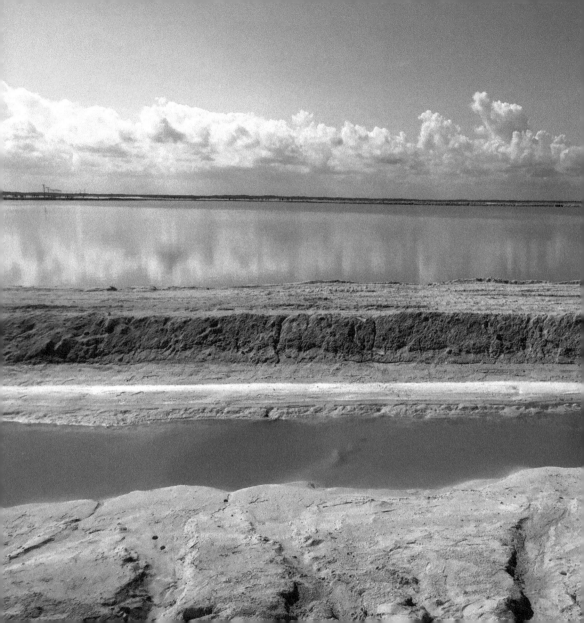

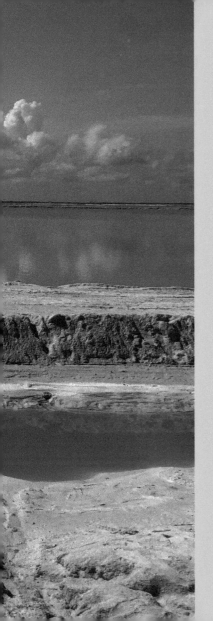

Little Ideas for July

Treat the Earth well.

Kenyan proverb

The whole of the Kenyan proverb on the last page goes as follows: '*Treat the Earth well. It was not given to you by your parents, it was loaned to you by your children.*' We can all do our part for the planet by thinking about what we use every day.

Micro-plastics from synthetic fabrics are a problem when they get into waste water, and we can avoid them by buying clothes made with natural materials like bamboo, hemp and organic cotton. We can support zero-waste stores which sell staple ingredients and cleaning products without plastic. We can also find creative re-uses for the plastic and other packaging we can't avoid. Here are some ideas for reducing or reusing plastic:

- Choose an ice-cream cone instead of opting for a paper cup and plastic spoon
- Buy some reusable beeswax food covers to use in place of plastic wrap

- Refill spray bottles with your own homemade surface cleaner, infusing one part water, one part white vinegar and some lemon rind
- Invest in a water bottle, reusable cup and straw and carry them with you

Look out too for clever initiatives such as Terracycle's Loop, which partners with major brands in the US, UK and Europe and is expanding. Loop delivers your shopping and collects the used containers with your next delivery, cleans them and returns them to the manufacturer for refill. ReturnR in Australia does the same with containers that restaurants use for collection or delivery.

Some tea bags contain polypropylene, a plastic used in sealing them shut. Look for plastic-free brands or switch to loose-leaf tea.

A society grows great when old men plant trees in whose shade they know they shall never sit.

Anonymous

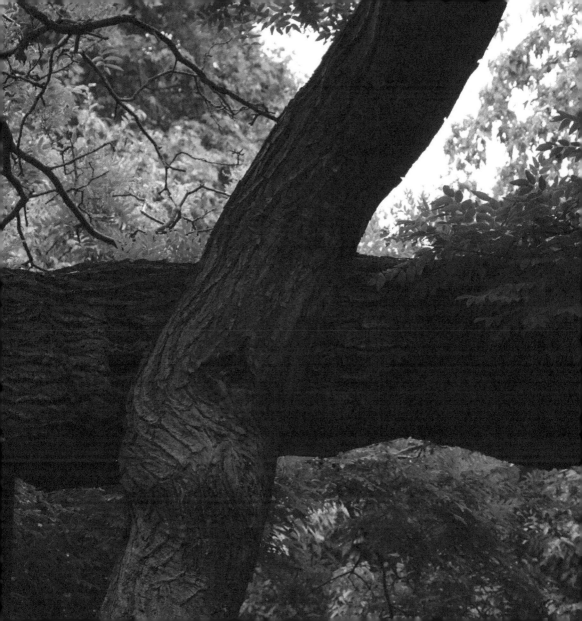

To encourage butterflies and other wildlife into your garden - or even a balcony or terrace - you just need to provide some food and water for them. Butterflies, bees and other pollinating insects love buddleja, verbena and hebe. Bees in particular like purple flowers, so lavender and alliums are good choices. To help a struggling bee, see p 44.

Wild birds will enjoy a shallow dish of water to drink and bathe in and will visit your garden more often if there is something for them to eat. While you can buy bird tables and special food, it's easy to make feeders at home.

Not doing some of the gardening can also help: leave your lawn unmown so that wildflowers like clover and buttercups appear.

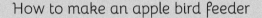

How to make an apple bird feeder

You will need:
An apple
An apple corer
A skewer
Sunflower seeds
Some thin sticks and string

Method:
Remove the core of the apple
Push the sunflower seeds into the top and sides of the apple
Make holes through the lower half of the apple with the skewer and
push the sticks through to make perches for the birds
Thread the string through the hole in the apple so you can hang up
your feeder

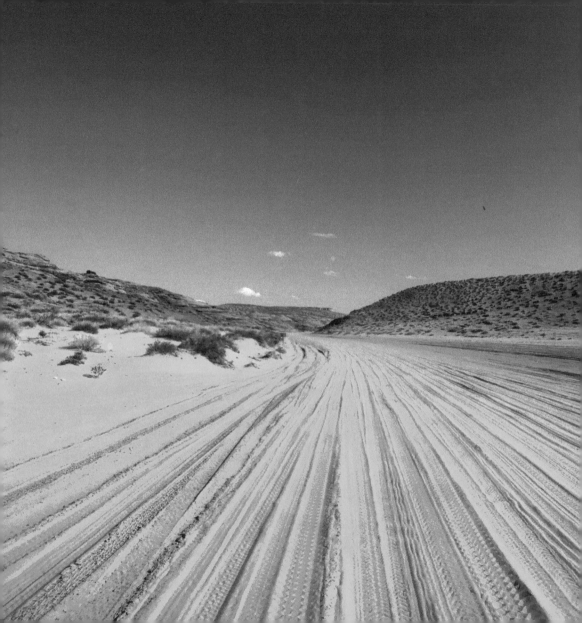

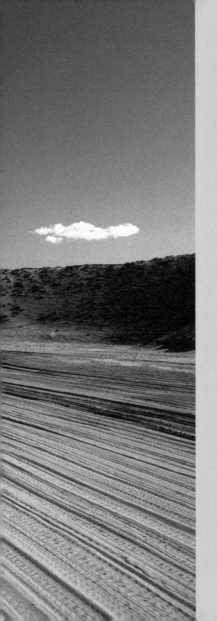

Little Ideas for August

Leave the road,
take the trails.

Pythagoras

While summer gives us the chance to spend more time out of doors relaxing, gardening or enjoying al-fresco meals, it can also be a good time to set yourself a new exercise goal.

A simple, brisk walk each day can bring all sorts of benefits, from strengthening bones and muscles, to improving balance and coordination, to lifting your mood. Aim for 30 minutes, or a couple of 15-minute walks, perhaps one in the morning and one after dinner, to take advantage of the light evenings.

Look for Tai Chi, dance and yoga classes in community parks or become a member of a local cycling group. There are also fun fitness challenges online. Some support a particular charity while others give the chance to experience an iconic journey virtually, at your own pace and without the cost of travelling around the world. We love these ideas for virtual challenges.

- Download an app like *Charity Miles* or *BetterPoints*. Your activity turns into donations for good causes

- Sign up online for a *Race at your Pace* challenge or a virtual walking route like the 480 mile *Camino de Santiago*. Reaching milestones on the journey triggers custom postcards and the planting of real trees

Researchers have found that being outside enhances mental as well as physical health, with test participants showing increased self-esteem and feelings of connection with nature and their community.

- If you'd like to take on a longer distance, organizers say that the *Walk 1000 Miles Challenge* can be completed in an hour a day over the course of a year

Fresh air impoverishes the doctor.

Danish proverb

Enjoying some fresh air can be a free and easy daily habit which brings us so many benefits. Studies show that there are physical and emotional advantages to spending time outside and that being in the open air, surrounded by nature, for just twenty minutes a day can increase energy and vitality by 90%.

To begin your day well, you can do something as simple as taking your first cup of tea or coffee to drink outdoors or even near an open window. Around a fifth of the oxygen you breathe in is needed by your brain to help it work at its best. Increased oxygen also improves the function of every cell in the body, benefitting the immune system, improving sleep quality, lowering blood pressure and reducing the stress hormone cortisol.

The weather may have other plans, of course, and that is when you can bring the outside in by adding some greenery to your home. Houseplants help purify and humidify the air and some also produce oxygen at night, making them good options for a bedroom. Your florist or nursery can help you make your choice, but some varieties to consider include:

- Orchids
- Succulents
- Bamboo palm
- Peace lilies
- Spider plants
- Gerbera daisies

Summer afternoon - to me these have always been the two most beautiful words in the English language.
Henry James

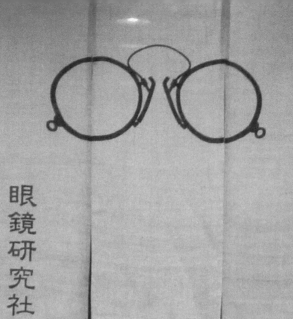

眼鏡研究社

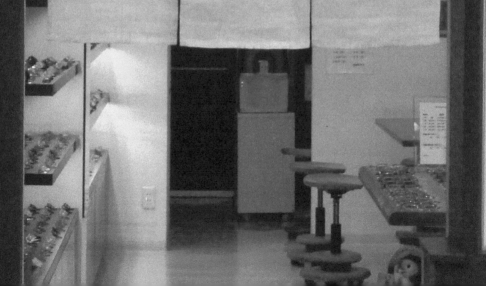

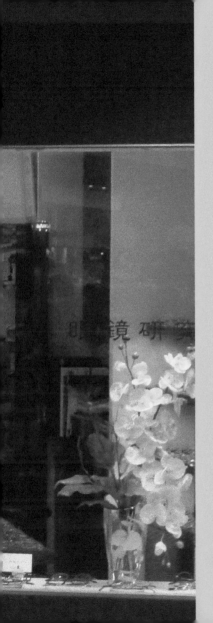

Little
Ideas
for
September

Reading is the key that
opens doors.

Ruth Bader Ginsburg

For many of us, September brings with it that 'back to school' feeling, so it's the perfect month to immerse yourself in something fresh to read, watch, listen to and learn. Here are some ideas for places online to explore and discover new things, all free of charge.

Futurelearn (futurelearn.com) offers hundreds of courses from universities and industry leaders all over the world. Topics range from the creative arts to science and engineering, as well as vocational subjects such as business, management and healthcare.

Ted Talks (ted.com) are given by experts in creativity, education, science, technology and design - covering everything from using paper towels more efficiently, to how money can buy happiness (depending on how you spend it). The mission of this organization is to spread ideas, with the core belief that ideas have the power to change attitudes, lives and ultimately, the world.

Duolingo (duolingo.com) is a great place to learn a new language, along with more than 1.2 billion others. Duolingo is rooted in the belief that learning a language can widen opportunity and mutual understanding.

Google Arts & Culture (artsandculture.google.com) is an amazing interactive gateway to galleries and museums worldwide. You can tour over 2000 museums, galleries and other cultural institutions via the website or by downloading the app.

Librivox (librivox.org) is a wonderful library of audiobooks. These are free recordings of books in the public domain, read by volunteers from across the world in all languages. If you feel inspired, you can get involved as a volunteer reader yourself.

Research has found that reading for just six minutes can reduce stress by 68%.

What on earth could be more luxurious
than a sofa, a book and a cup of coffee?

Anthony Trollope

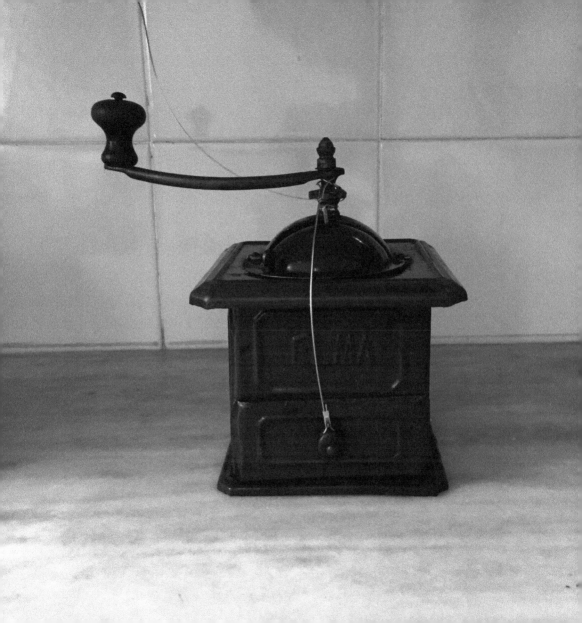

Since September marks the beginning of the harvest, what better time to make good use of all you have learned in a fun way that tests your knowledge and helps others in need of food.

Free Rice (freerice.com) is an online general knowledge quiz from the United Nations World Food Programme. For every correct answer, a sponsored advert generates money for grains of rice to feed the hungry, and to enable education for children who would otherwise go without nourishment.

Free Rice is just one of many games that promote change, education, skills development and social innovation. You can find a collection of over 175 games on the website **Games for Change** (gamesforchange.org), which helps to empower game designers to improve communities and drive social change, in order to make the world a better place.

International Literacy Day is also celebrated in September. The World Literacy Foundation runs a series of special events this month to promote literacy in communities around the world. Here are some ways to get involved:

- Volunteer at a local library, reading club or story telling group
- Support a charity that promotes literacy with donations of books or money for learning resources and teaching materials
- Share and promote International Literacy Day on social media

Reading is a passport to countless adventures.

Mary Pope Osborne

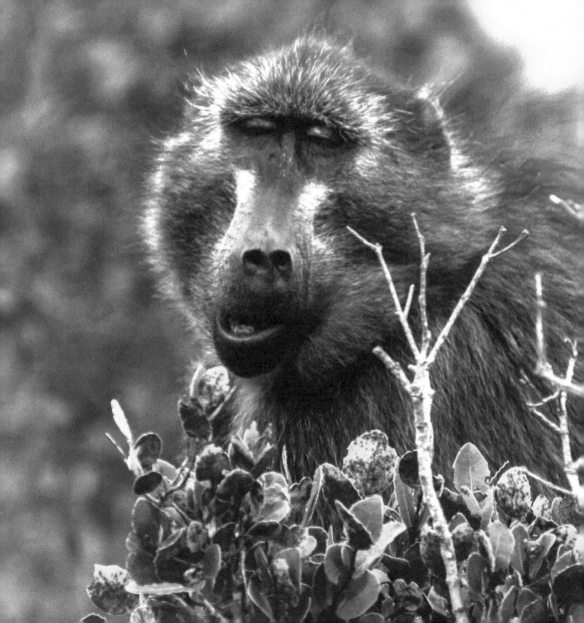

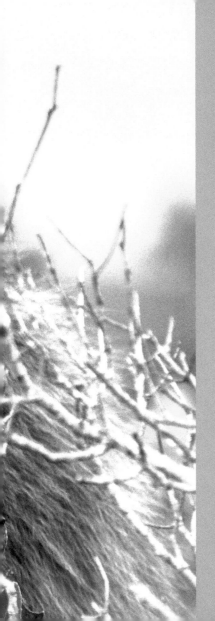

Little Ideas for October

Everyone smiles in the
same language.

George Carlin

October begins with World Smile Day, when we're all called upon to do one act of kindness that makes one person smile. It doesn't matter how small that act of kindness seems; perhaps it is simply holding the door open for someone, or paying a compliment, or calling a loved one, or lending a helping hand.

Sometimes that act of kindness is smiling itself – lifting someone else's mood and making their life a little happier. And then, because smiling is contagious, the effect goes on, and someone else's life is happier in turn.

A wise grandfather once said, 'if your face wants to smile, let it; and if it doesn't, make it'. In other words, be mindful, and even if you don't feel like smiling, do so consciously, because the very act of smiling can bring you all sorts of benefits.

- Smiling triggers the release of neurotransmitters like dopamine, which act as natural anti-depressants

- Smiling helps you relax, lowering your blood pressure and helping your immune system function more effectively

- The muscles you use to smile lift your face and make you appear more confident and more youthful

- Smiling helps you to stay positive - it's hard to smile and think negatively at the same time

The Anglo-Saxons called October wyn-monath or wine month, the time that the grapes were harvested and pressed. A very good reason to smile!

We shall never know all the good that a simple smile can do.

Mother Teresa

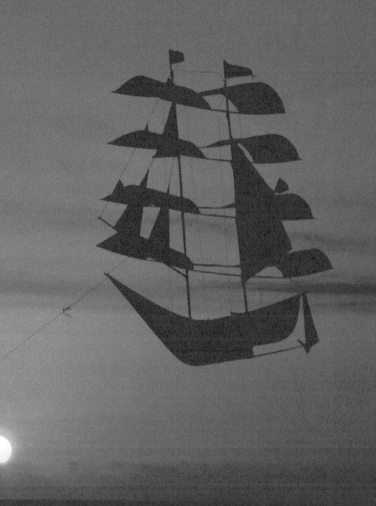

Here are some things that make us smile this time of year, and we hope you might set aside some time to enjoy a few of them too:

- Taking a moment to marvel at the warm and wonderful hues of autumn leaves
- Heading to the park and swooshing around in piles of fallen leaves
- Going for a bike ride
- Picking apples. Baking apple pies or crisps or crumbles
- Visiting the pumpkin farm
- Carving jack-o-lanterns
- Making warming casseroles and soups
- Digging out your cosiest sweater
- Playing board games
- Stocking up on cinnamon and other warming spices

- Looking up at the stars on a cold, crisp night
- Making a playlist to greet trick-or-treaters on Hallowe'en. Some of our most-loved are classic tracks from *Harry Potter*, *Ghostbusters*, *The Addams Family*, *The Rocky Horror Picture Show* and *Thriller*
- Gathering around a fire and toasting marshmallows
- Snuggling up with a good novel and a mug of hot chocolate (or hot spiced apple cider – see p 92)
- Going back to much-loved children's book or TV show: nothing beats *Winnie the Pooh* or *The Land of Green Ginger* or *It's the Great Pumpkin, Charlie Brown*

I'm so glad I live in a world where there are Octobers.
LM Montgomery, *Anne of Green Gables*

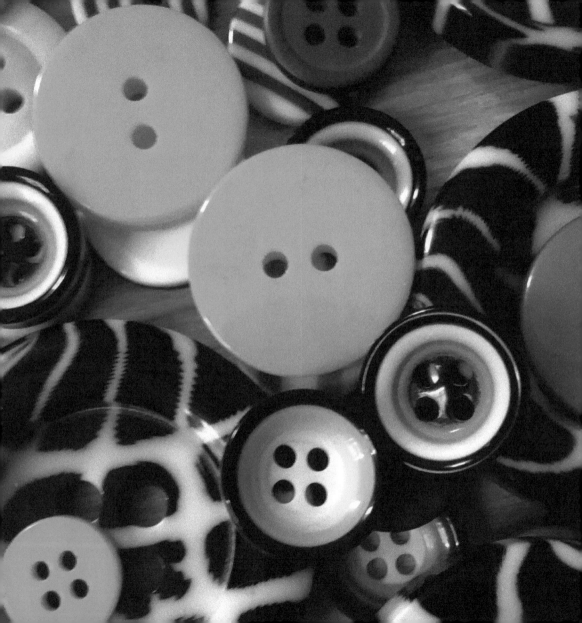

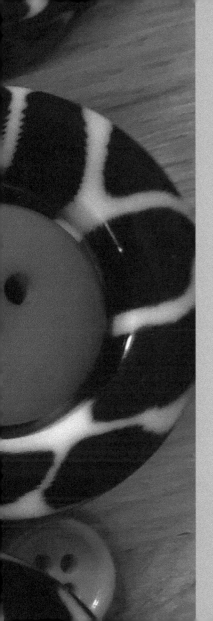

Little Ideas for November

Be present in all things and
thankful for all things.

Maya Angelou

Here we are in November. The harvest season is coming to a close and the evenings are drawing in. Before we get caught up in the bustle of the holiday season, it is a good time to relax and breathe deeply; to reflect on the past year and for all those things for which we are thankful.

Relax and breathe deeply
Spending just a few minutes each day to concentrate on your breathing can slow your heart rate and promote physical, mental and spiritual well-being. *Susokukan*, Japanese for counting the breath with numbers, is a Buddhist practice that helps you focus and relax.

- Sit in a comfortable position
- Close your eyes if you like
- Breathe... counting your exhales
- If your mind wanders and you get distracted, simply start again
- Try this for just ten minutes and feel the effect of calm

Reflect and be grateful

One simple way to do this is to keep a journal. Again this need not be an arduous process, and it has so many benefits. A recent study demonstrated that people who wrote down three things for which they were grateful over the course of one week, and identified the causes of those good things, felt an increased sense of happiness even six months later. Or if you prefer not to write, just be deliberate: each night when you brush your teeth, for example, make a habit of calling to mind something for which you are grateful. Both will brighten your smile!

Frankincense promotes a sense of gratitude and peace. Diffuse by itself or blend with bergamot and lavender.

Let us be grateful to the people who make us happy; they are the charming gardeners who make our souls blossom.

Marcel Proust

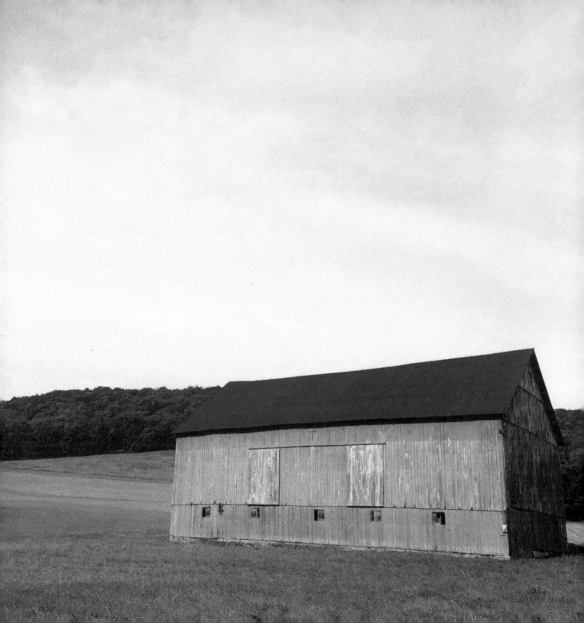

HOT SPICED APPLE CIDER

Warming drinks tinged with spices and sugars are perfect for celebrations this time of year. As an alternative to classic mulled wine – which the Romans created back in the 2nd century to help them keep warm in freezing winters – try a hot spiced apple cider. Delicious paired with some tangy blue cheese, sausage rolls, mini croque monsieurs or for an entirely sweet treat, some warm cinnamon sugar doughnuts.

Ingredients
4 cups (1000 ml) apple juice or cider
1 cinnamon stick, broken into pieces
¼ teaspoon of cloves
2 star anise
3-4 slices of fresh orange and lemon
3 thin slices of fresh ginger root

Method
Mix everything together in a large saucepan
Cover and heat gently until the mixture starts to steam, then leave for 15 minutes to infuse
If you'd like a little extra sweetness, add brown sugar to taste
Remove the fruit and spices with a slotted spoon and serve, garnished with slices of apple

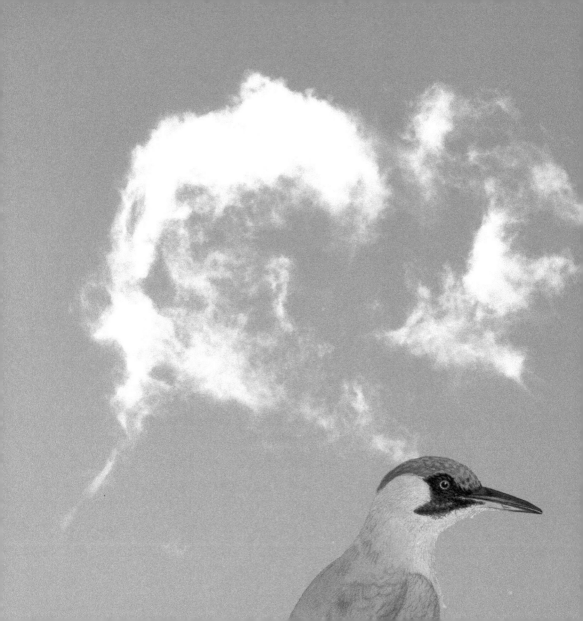

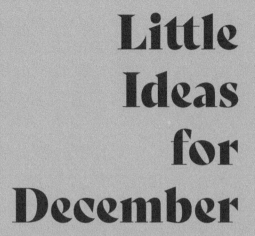

Little Ideas for December

Kindness is generally reciprocal.

Dr Samuel Johnson

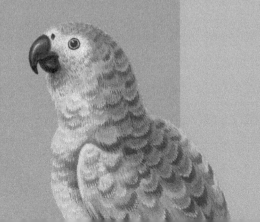

It is the season of goodwill. Whether your tradition is Christmas, Hanukkah or Kwaanza, or you just enjoy this time of year, it's a time of light and hope and giving to others. And it's full of anticipation.

Anticipation is embodied in Advent and the giving of Advent calendars. There are several nice calendar concepts to make your countdown more meaningful. We love these ideas, for adults and children:

- Kindness calendars. These suggest a kind deed each day: you can print one from the Action for Happiness website, actionforhappiness.org, or you might find one in the store that also includes delicious chocolate rewards.

- Giving calendars. These contain a pack of craft supplies each day to make a gift for someone else

- Reverse advent calendars. Reverse because you put something in each day, rather than take something out; and at the end of advent (or a few days before) you have a collection of food, or clothing, or toys to take to a local charity and help a family in need enjoy a happier holiday

December 6th is the Feast of St Nicholas, who was noted for his generosity in helping children, the poor and those in need. Among the traditions for celebrating the day is the giving of gifts in shoes or stockings. Over time, St Nicholas has become associated with Santa Claus and the bringing of gifts to children all over the world.

Gifts of time and love are surely the
ingredients of a truly merry Christmas.

Peg Bracken

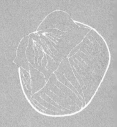

Roast chestnuts

As the lights begin twinkling in the windows and the snow starts to flurry, chestnut sellers appear at holiday markets or on street corners with their braziers and their blackened paper bags of steaming hot chestnuts. Here is a simple recipe for a treat at home.

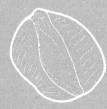

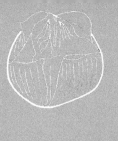

Preheat the oven to 200C/400F

Carefully cut an x on the flat side of each
nut, using a sharp paring knife
Lay the chestnuts, x-side up, in a single
layer on a baking sheet
Roast for about 30 minutes
Cool, peel and enjoy

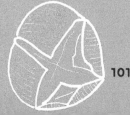

I felt once more how simple and frugal a
thing is happiness: a glass of wine,
a roast chestnut, a wretched little brazier,
the sound of the sea.

Nikos Kazantzakis

We wish you every happiness, and a life lived well.

Photos by Cristina

CPSIA information can be obtained
at www.ICGtesting.com
Printed in the USA
BVHW021341020621
608650BV00003B/254